Look at

How I did it...

MY WEIGHT LOSS
JOURNEY

Authored by: S. T. Williams

Table of Contents

Chapter 1

Getting Started: My Weight Loss History

When I first had the idea of wanting to lose weight, the thought of a new challenge was what made me anticipate the end results. It was high school, when I first decided that it was time for me to change. High school might seem like it was too early to think about my weight, but I was not super skinny at all, in fact I was around, 187 pounds, 5 feet 7 inches. Having the overweight appearance, was not cool, but I am a person that would not sit around, so I did something about it. During that time, I wanted to find something that could burn fat, but I really didn't know what I was looking for, I knew that I wanted to lose weight, fast and quick.

During my search, I found, diet pills that I thought were going to help burn the fat off. I picked up the bottle and read the directions, a program was described on the bottle as: thirty days to burn fat along with diet and exercise. At first, it seemed as if I had lost hope, but I found something that would help burn the fat off, I did, in thirty days, just like the directions instructed. I had to think about the situation, nothing is permanent, at some point maintenance will be needed, and with taking those pills everyday was not something that I wanted to do. I mean really, not that many people love to take huge oval shaped pills that get stuck in the throat.

Later, I began to feel like I still couldn't eat what I wanted, well at least food that taste good, but portioned out in the right amounts. Not knowing how to portion out my own food really hindered my weight loss progress. While taking the pills I ate many salads with ranch dressing topping, and that did not help me lose the weight that I was looking to lose. I'm thinking, because the dressing was high in fat, also not knowing the right amount of lettuce, and lastly what to put on the salad was also a problem. There were other foods that I ate thinking that I was eating right but just not the right portion size. Running, salads, and diet pills combined was beneficial, because I lost around 10 pounds in about 30 days.

Well here I go, I really thought that was something, but I did lose weight with the diet pills just not enough weight in thirty days. When I looked at my body I felt like there was still more weight that needed to be taken off. I thought that maybe I needed to lose around twenty more pounds. At that point I was still in the need of searching for the right thing that could give me what I was looking for.

While researching many different products and strategies for weight loss it can become time consuming and challenging, but it was important for me to find exactly what I needed. The search was on when it came to looking for that one thing, I just knew I would find something to help me lose that twenty pounds, trust me I searched. One day, I was watching TV a commercial for a weight loss program popped up. This commercial gave instructions on how to call in, get started, and lose nineteen pounds in twenty days. (I think this was what the commercial described, it has been a while, and I have not seen that program commercial currently, please don't quote me on that exactly.) Anyhow, I called up that company and said to them, "I want to sign up with their weight loss program." I ended up traveling about thirty minutes a week to try this program out for those days specified.

The program consisted of daily portioned out food that was purchased from the company's store, a food diary that contained some information on what foods that can be added to the plan, space to keep track of the daily food intake, and some other pamphlets. The program required, to follow a constructed meal plan and eat those portioned out foods added with exercise; there for, losing the pounds in twenty days, but I didn't think that sounded to promising and unrealistic. During my time on that program it became very interesting to me, switching to more manageable portioned out foods and having a meal plan to go off of. I kept up exercise and stuck with the meal plan for the twenty days, it seemed to had worked for me; what I am saying is that I did lose twenty pounds in twenty days, and I was shocked, but very excited that I finally lost some more weight. I wanted to continue on with this program, but without buying the foods directly from the company, I decided to buy the same foods, but from a grocery store.

Continuing on with the program without the company's foods, but foods from the grocery store, I purchased the same foods just cheaper. I had learned what portion size to use, because of the information that was in the food diary the weight loss company provided me. Something happened while I continued that program, first, I got bored with eating those same foods. The foods were good, but I had the same thing over and over, and got bored it made me uninterested. Second, doing the same workout, my body reacted to that and stopped showing any results. There was no more weight loss, it just stopped, and it was almost like I was just maintaining my weight instead of losing weight. At that time, I had no idea about plateaus, and no idea of how to lose body fat, all I knew is that I wanted to achieve my goal, get the weight off, and fast.

This started a new journey, it was a long one, on the road to a successful weight loss. During that period there was nothing left for me to do, I thought that maybe there was nothing out there that would help me continue to lose weight, to become what I wanted to see every day. This course ran over for years and years of trying to lose weight with just portion control. I became interested in the diet pills then following the weight loss program, I soon realized after the baby that I really needed to get those pounds off or they would stick around for the rest of my life.

My mother is obese; when she was in high school she was the total opposite; she was a smaller girl wearing a size five. After my mother had her first child which was I, she lost weight and had a shape to her body. Then my mother had her second child and that's when she gained much weight and couldn't or didn't know how to take the weight off, so over the years she became obese. Since I could remember, I had struggled up and down with my weight and nothing stood out as noticeable weight loss. Then, I didn't want to give up, because I am a determined person, but I was lost and didn't know what to do or how to get the weight off.

As I continued my search, I came across a gym; it was a new gym in my area that consisted of, thirty second interval exercise circuits. When I came across this gym, I became excited all over again, because it was something new, that I had not tried before. Well, the next day I went to the gym, signed up, and couldn't wait to begin my workout. I noticed right away that the place was very bright in yellow colors along with the exercise machines, that looked so foreign to me. Then, there was a space for shoes and coats, but I couldn't believe the quaint space, and no locker rooms. Lastly, right before I had entered the area with exercise equipment, there was the receptionist desk, a tall semicircular desk painted gray and white in color. I was excited and overwhelmed at the same time, because I was hoping for some sort of miracle at this point.

No turning back, first day of workout I noticed this board on the wall, it supposed to be some sort of motivation for the gym members. It consisted of members' weight loss in a week, it also showed others who got praise for losing weight every week. Going to the gym would had been my first time at using any exercise machine like those, and it appeared as it would had been hard to do, but it was a good thing the staff showed the members how to do the exercises and properly use equipment. That day, I started on the first machine in rotation, as the music played there was a thirty second indicator that alerted when it was time to switch to the next machine. I believed, I did the complete circuit around a few sessions in about thirty minutes' time. After the workout that day, I felt really good and energized, and anticipated going back to the gym the next day. By the way, the staff was very nice and helpful, suggested that members come around three to four times a week to complete the circuit in thirty minutes. Well, that really didn't sound all that bad, three to four times a week in just thirty minutes, I felt like I could definitely do that with no problem. I was concerned to see some results, but I wanted to see them fast. Going to that gym was fun for the first three weeks, because it was something new that I had not tried and hoped that I would see some results.

After going to that gym my first week I lost around twelve pounds, I felt great, I was then placed on the board for that week weight loss. My second week there, I lost around three pounds, and third week is when I lost around one to two pounds. Now of course, I was so happy that first week, because I lost twelve pounds and that's what gave me motivation to continue to go back to the gym. By the staff placing my weight loss on the board, it gave me motivation to continue to go back, but at the end of the second week I

couldn't believe I had only lost three pounds. That may sound

good to some, but for me that was not what I was looking for. I

think that going to that gym was the slowest process ever, to

lose one to three pounds a week, it would have taken me

forever to achieve what I wanted to accomplish. After the third

week, I didn't feel motivated to continue there, I felt like the

weight had stop coming off, and I was stuck yet again. I found

all sorts of excuses to get out of that program, just so I could

cancel my membership. Soon that situation was over and I

was on my search again, but then I began to procrastinate on

looking for ways to lose weight because I became

unmotivated.

By becoming unmotivated, it kind of put a hold on my

search, even though I knew I should had been doing some

sort of workout, but sometimes things take a back seat. At that

point of my life, I was still trying to get the fat off, that was all I

could think about. One thing I did learn during that process

was, it's hard to get that thick layer of fat off the belly. I decided

to snap out of it, because I didn't want that big belly remaining a lingering problem, that was something that I did not want, so I did something about it.

I began trying different things to lose weight, such as protein shakes, lemonade detox, and soup diets. I didn't understand what a protein shake was at that point, all I knew was to drink a shake in the place of a meal, as so I thought. Protein shakes did not work for me, it made me gain weight, and I was hungry all the time, I didn't know how to use those shakes properly. I tried an all soup diet, and that didn't go well, because I was always hungry with that. I had tried the lemonade detox, with cayenne pepper and maple syrup, but I was extremely hungry with that one also.

Over the years I kept trying diets that never worked, or I lost maybe one to two pounds and after a few weeks no more weight loss. After a while had past, I began running around in my neighborhood as some form of exercise, then one day watching TV I came across this DVD exercise program. I ordered the program, it came in the mail, inside was, DVDs, meal plan, recipes, and a two-month calendar with scheduled exercises for specified days. During the first month workouts were six day workouts, but the second month got even harder, it also was six days a week.

At the beginning of the first month, I worked out six days a week, and followed the meal plan as instructed. I noticed right away, that I didn't need to buy much food, the meal plan was very simple and easy to follow. The workouts were very hard in the beginning, but I pushed through it. By the end of the third week, I began to get custom to the workouts, and it became easier. When I began the second month, workouts became much harder and longer sessions. I kept up with the meal plan and the six-day workout schedule. I also finished that DVD program in sixty days, saw a difference, I was much more toned up than before, but nowhere near my ideal look because I was still over weight. I really enjoyed that DVD program, it was very challenging and I learned so much. There was a lot of education in that DVD program, it helped me to figure out how excessing worked, along with eating the right foods and protein.

I guess I am a picky person, but I want it to count if I am doing it, that DVD program gave me a huge boost in the exercise department. Well, I must say that when performing those exercises, they were not easy, but I went at my own speed in the beginning, but eventually I developed strength to push myself harder and harder each time. I learned to take control of my eating habits, and I was brought to another level of thinking when it came to working out. Doing crunches on the floor is one thing I hate, but that program taught me how to do abdominal workouts standing up, it was amazing.

The meal plan was great, because it gave me a variety of choices for five meals a day. The recipes to those meals included nutritional information that helped for me to know exactly how many calories and other nutritional information I needed. Some of these weight loss programs won't tell how many calories are in certain meals let alone tell how to calculate your own daily calorie intake. Not knowing how to calculate the number of calories to eat for my body type and weight was something I never knew how to do before. Learning those simple things can go a long way in the future, because it offered a foundation to start from.

There were some cons with that DVD program, such as the long workouts, which lasted anywhere between, thirty to forty-five minutes each session. It was very hard sometimes to get sixty minutes in for a workout and sometimes it was hard to get in any workout at all. Working out was and is, a very essential part of losing weight, the foods I ate really affected the outcome of those daily workouts. Those simple tools that I learned, I plan on using all of them in a combination of my own meal plan and workout schedule to lose the weight. My next challenge would be to lose the weight successfully and discover a new way of living. That new way of living would consist of a much cleaner eating, and exercise that would help for future success in weight loss.

Chapter 2

Losing the Weight: Finding a Plan that Works for me

I utilized my motivation and determination, to begin with designed a meal plan and exercise schedule. In the beginning of this journey, I definitely started off wrong with the food choices, along with different programs to lose weight. For me, there are very little items that I will eat, which will have benefits my body needs for fuel and energy purposes. I didn't want to eat for no purpose, such as: eating because someone else is eating, bored, stressed, and just see items to eat that look appetizing. I was eating salads I thought would help me lose weight, when it actually did nothing to help aid in my weight loss. Items like, soup diets and pills, all that stuff I tried, I truly thought those things were going to work, but unfortunately they didn't. Well those things did not exceed my expectations in the weight loss area that I was looking for.

With that being said, those were the reasons I found my own way of losing the weight. This is not something that I am saying will work for someone else, but it worked for me, some things that work for others may not work for another person. This is why I call it *My Journey to weight loss...,* because it's my perspective on how I lost my weight.

The meal plan was very simple to design, as it follows more than a diet it's a way of eating foods that produce results (I will frequently refer to this detox meal plan as Phase 1). On that first week, I weighed in over two hundred pounds, that weight alone gave me motivation to get started. As I began the first three to four days, I was extremely hungry, but determined to keep pushing through. Here are examples and variety of ways on how each day went for me until I lost the desired amount of weight.

At the beginning of day one (Phase 1), I gathered, a variety of fruit (e.g. apples and oranges), a gallon of water, and some walnuts. Starting in the morning with my favorite extra-large bowl, like a mixing bowl used to mix a cake in. Chopped up all the fruit then place inside the bowl it does not matter what kind of fruit, it can be the same fruit, or it can be all different kinds of fruits. Next is to get a small separate container for nuts, I only put around a cup of walnuts in my container per day, it must be walnuts, only because they were the most filling for me, and lastly, the gallon of water. I could have refilled the bowl many times a day, but I did not refill my

bowl with fruit.

All day whenever I felt hungry I ate fruit out of my bowl,

some of the nuts throughout the day, and also drank water

throughout the day until all gone. At the end of the day there

was no fruit, no nuts, and no water left, I repeated that process

over again on day two, and kept repeating daily until the

desired weight loss.

Now here are the other ways to do this same meal plan

- take all of your favorite vegetables and only steam cook. Do

not add these items: No salt, No seasonings, No butter, No

added seasonings with salt, but herbs, garlic, black pepper

that's it. Fill up the mixing bowl with the steamed veggies, get

a half of a cup of walnuts in a separate container, and get a

gallon of water for the day. Eat off of the veggies, eat the half

of a cup of walnuts and drink the water all day until all gone.

Another variation would be to fill the mixing bowl up and eat

fruits and steamed veggies, half a cup of walnuts, and drink

the gallon of water all day.

Here are my rules: eat all the fruits and veggies I wanted all day long even late at night, drink the gallon of water or more daily, only eat the recommended amount of walnuts a day since they are higher in fat, no pop, no candy, no seasonings with sodium, only use salt free herbs, garlic, and black pepper - no salt, no meat, no alcohol, no bread, no crackers, no sweets, chewing sugarless gum was ok, no fast food, no sit down and eat restaurants, not nothing, but what's on this meal list (Table 1), no white potatoes, no yellow potatoes, sweet potatoes are the only potatoes, all veggies and fruits except anything I have mentioned not to eat. Here is a full view of the list of foods (Table 1) that cannot be eaten and a list of the foods I could eat. Sometimes showing items in a different way may help to understand the food list.

My Food List (Phase 1)

Foods Not to Eat	Foods to Eat
Sugar (all types)	
Bread (all types)	
Salt	
Pineapples (high in sugar)	
Seasoning Salt	
All Salt based Seasonings	
White Potatoes	
Yellow Potatoes	
Red Potatoes	
Pop	
Candy	Sweet Potatoes (only)
Junk Foods (chips, cakes, pies, ice cream, popsicle, donuts, candy bars)	Any Fruit, Limitless (example: Oranges and apples)
Meat (all types and forms)	Limit the number of Grapes daily (14 Grapes)
Condiments (ketchup, salt, mustard, relish, mayo, mayonnaise)	Herbs
Oil (all types)	Black Pepper
Cereal	Salt Free Seasonings
Salads	Vegetables, Limitless (all, except those potatoes on the not to eat list)
Fast Food (exceptions are fruit plates and steamed vegetables, no salt based seasonings)	
Fat Free Foods	
Low Sodium Foods	
Diet Drinks	
Artificial Flavors	
Preservatives	
Processed Foods	
High Fructose Corn Syrup	
Syrup	

Table 1

*Motivational Tip: Try not to get to discouraged, my food list is something I am sharing with you. I found motivation during (**Phase 1**), my motivation was determination and a picture of Beyoncé. As you can see that it does not matter what type of motivation you have just have some, it is important to keep going, push hard every day, and to stay focused. It will not happen overnight, but over time the results will become more amazing.

Things to Recap (Phase 1)

- ✓ Eat fruit and/or veggies all day
- ✓ Nuts
- ✓ I ate fruit up into late night if hungry
- ✓ Drink gallon of water daily (Minimum limit)
- ✓ Stayed away from the foods on not to eat list (See Table 1)
- ✓ Didn't exercise – not yet

My Daily Water Intake (Phase 1)

A gallon of water = 128 oz. / 3.78 liters

My water bottle weight = 1.05 qt. / 1 litter / 33.6 oz.

My total amount of water using my designated bottle = 4

bottles / 33.6 oz. bottle / 132 oz.

Chapter 3

Motivation

Motivation is very important not only at this phase, but it really helps when things seem to get too tough. For me, this food plan was harder the first few days, it became challenging by the fifth day, but by the seventh day things got better, I became more adaptive to the food plan. In my mind, I thought about how much I wanted to lose weight and how long of a journey it had been. Determination helped me to become more focused on what the goal was, and my future outcome.

Within the first two weeks my body began to get rid of all those annoying toxins that had permitted an extreme hold on weight loss. I continued the meal plan (Table 1), stayed focused on jumpstarting the weight loss and not so much focus on the weight loss time frame. The time spent during (Phase 1) was not calculated, but it was monitored. While beginning (Phase 1) many will think that I stayed on track the whole time, but reality is I am human, and, yes I did slack a few times here and there. It's ok to have days where slacking off is ok, but I didn't make this a habit. I gave myself once a week was the max for slacking off, because the rest of the week was available for redemption, since I needed motivation for sweets cravings. My body began to want things that normally there was no craving for; such as sweets, this is how the body works and it's all in the mind, trust me. This was the hardest stage (Phase 1), the body was basically preparing to rebuild itself by: getting rid of toxins from social alcohol drinking, fatty red meat, junk food, unhealthy oils, and other toxins, all to enhance the metabolism.

Many people will try to discourage or make many comments on what your body needs to lose weight, listen to the body, and if there are medical conditions or diabetes present this may not be for that type of person. Rapid weight loss has positive effects that's, fast weight loss results, and, also negative effects, that's lose skin and no muscle tone. Remember I have been overweight for majority of my life there will be loose skin. This is nothing to fear as everyone is different and the most common area for loose skin is breast, arms, abdominal, and thighs. The most noticeable loose skin will be in the front abdominal area, and this just depends on the person not everyone.

Motivation, it can come from many areas of your life, and provide just what is needed to succeed. I am motivation to many individuals since my weight loss, because of the amazing transformation results I had with this method. The purpose of this book is to: tell what I did to lose weight, and what were the methods that I designed to produce weight loss. During (Phase 1) I did not do any exercise during that period, because I was trying to melt off some of that fat first before adding exercise such as, strength training and weight lifting. One thing I never starved my body, because it would have had to use the muscles as an energy source (this means loss of muscle). There would have been a constant demand for food if I was exercising and performing (Phase 1), the body would burn those natural sugars up quickly, at that point, my body would be hungry, and therefore not enough of nutrients and protein needed to sustain a workout.

Prior to (Phase 1) I was eating many processed foods that caused heart burn, foods that had my belly bloated, foods that had too much sodium, and mainly everything I ate did not help me to lose weight. Since the cleansing of toxins, through eating only fruits and vegetables, I have no heart burn issues, and I still maintain a new tailored food plan for my body. Even with that, there are some foods I still cannot consume such as some fruits, vegetables, milk, tomatoes, and as much as I love garlic, it's a culprit also. It took me a few months to lose some weight with (Phase 1,) but I saw results immediately and it was worth the time and effort that was put into this.

Motivation, it can go a long way when there are so many things that can discourage a person from losing weight, and obtaining a goal. In the beginning when my appearance changed people wanted to know was I, "sick" or "stressed out," because of my amazing transformation. Well, of course not, is the thought of wanting to be in shape and healthier than previous, too much to ask for? No, because I have always been healthy and exercised, it was not until now, that I had decided to take things to another level. Friends and family can say negative things, but never say, "congratulations on the weight loss," it's the stranger that will give the compliment. People I know have said that I'm to "...skinny," "...did I lose some more weight," "well, how much weight are you trying to lose?" Now, these things are said, sarcastically in effort to make me feel like I need to gain weight. I laugh, because in my opinion there is no way I looked better, overweight, than slim. Family would give invitations to events where the menu has food that is not healthy, meanwhile fixing a plate of food that's perceived as servings sized for a one-year-old, gives off the wrong perception. Please, don't believe that you are better than someone else just because of a plate size; I would rather have that smaller portion than an oversized portioned plate of food.

What I have learned in my opinion is, the main point of motivation is to have it for yourself, but not worry about if others motivate or support certain decisions. Push yourself to go workout, with a set out plan, eat healthy as often as possible but, remember certain things that are healthy can be bad if the amount eaten is large. Don't be afraid of the measuring cups, there is no way of knowing how much food that had been consumed, if measuring is not done. It's very simple to measure out food, in fact I recommend getting a scale for measuring lean meats and measuring cups for liquids, and other items, these will come in handy. There is no need to worry about being hungry, because eating small meals with equally high protein throughout the day will help keep the energy up and water helps keep a full feeling. Know how much exercise, food, protein, and fat intake daily the body needs to achieve a goal.

Chapter 4

Transformation

At this stage, I began to look at how much weight I had lost, my perception in the mirror confirmed how hard I had worked for the past months. Very determined, and eager to begin exercising, I developed my own workout circuits and meal plan. The workouts and meal plans were optimized for my body weight to ensure the best results. Before beginning my exercise routine, I determined my starting body weight, calculated daily water intake, calorie intake, protein and fat intake, and the type of food to eat. All those things are very important to know, but this is very simple to do because there are various websites that show how to do these simple calculations for free.

I began the second phase by exercising seven days a week in the gym. Starting with cardio (cardio is anything that gets the heart rate up), in my workouts I began off slow the first month, building my heart rate up to its max and keeping it there. Monitoring my rate was very important to know if I was pushing myself too hard with little effort or not pushing myself hard enough with the most effort. The body can be a weird machine so some days it will feel as if the body is weaker than other days, so keep an eye on how much protein the body gets so it can recover from intense workouts. My cardio sessions lasted around an hour each day that I worked out, during that hour I pushed myself to go harder each time and to challenge myself further.

I used the treadmill a lot during that first month then slowly moved my way into the next month doing HIIT, (High Intensity Interval Training) sessions. These sessions are very intense, a lot of sweat involved. Getting the heart rate up to its max and keeping it there for a certain amount of time, then decrease the heart rate by jogging or walking all while on the treadmill. I did intervals of one-minute-high max limit then, decrease 30 second jog, I would repeat this for up to ten minutes each HIIT session. HIIT burns fat all day long, it's very advanced but it can be done in any intervals and at your own pace, with different exercises. I kept this up for about two more months then it was time to switch things up since I really needed a lot of toning to do.

Strength training was the next thing I began working on because it adds definition to the muscles and brings a challenge to my workout. Now training at six days a week, eating clean meals daily, watching my calorie, fat, water, and protein intake. It was hard work, but it all payed off at the end and I don't regret it at all. Working out for at least an hour a day helped me get in a good sweat, while isolating each muscle group with increased weight each week and pushing further and further every week. Weight lifting never got burned out, only with repetitive usage of the same weight.

Protein is good for the body that's why I calculated my protein intake based off of my body weight and made sure I worked out hard on those days which are called the high days. High days are high protein days and low days are low protein days, more calories are burned on high protein days with the right amount of exercise. On those low days of course less calories are burned this is usually a rest day.

Eating clean, this is similar to the foods in (Table 1), but now meat (Chicken) is added, beans, brown rice, vegetables, and a few other food items back into my diet. It's not hard to find a clean food list online these days, which includes what foods and amounts are ok. I normally eat clean during training only because it gets boring after a while, but like I said I stayed focused. Eating chicken breast, a vegetable, natural peanut butter, some fruits and nuts are about a normal day's meal during training, but don't forget my protein shakes. Basically it's much easier to have my meals planned out daily in food containers, this way I stay on track with eating clean. All I did was pick out foods that I could tolerate on a daily basis and foods that were easy and quick to fix from the clean food list (similar to table 1). I was not about to spend hundreds, yet thousands of dollars on a trainer, a nutritionist, so doing my own research was very important to me, I put in a lot of work into maintaining this new look.

I keep the weight off very simple, and that's working out at least five to six days a week. It all depends on key factors such as age, weight, and activity level these are the things that I used to determine how many days of a week I should be more active. I must be active at least five days a week if I am not training and six days during training. At least five days a week will keep my weight maintained with food management, and portion control, but for me this means weighing and measuring everything. Weighing and measuring everything to maintain, that is the answer to the questions, for everyone who has asked me, "Why do you still work out?" and "How little are you trying to get?" All this seems like a diet, but for me it's a lifestyle, a way of life that feels awesome. I work hard at achieving different goals every six weeks, I will never stop going and I love it.

Second Phase Recap

- ✓ After detox fat loss
- ✓ Hit Gym, Eat clean, Four months' cardio workouts
- ✓ Begin strength training
- ✓ Calculate calorie intake
- ✓ Calculate protein intake
- ✓ Met all six week goals

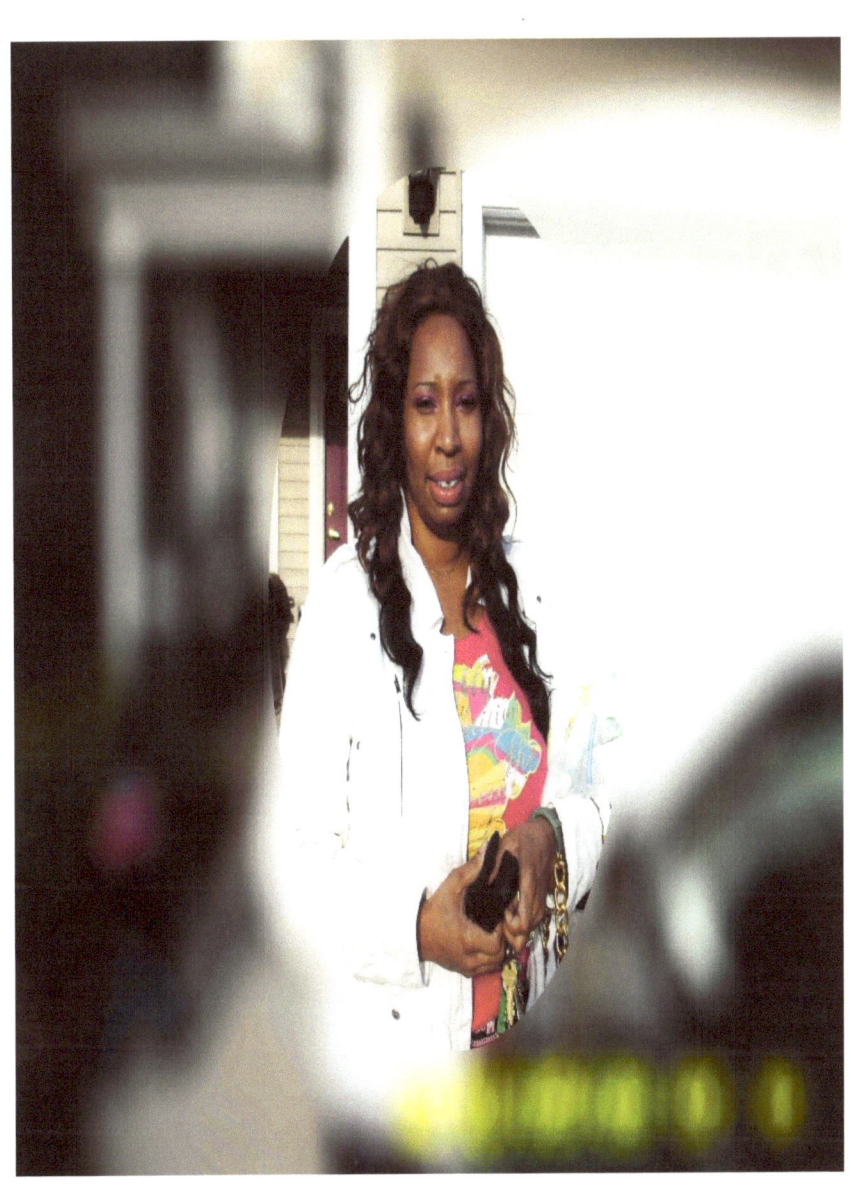

35

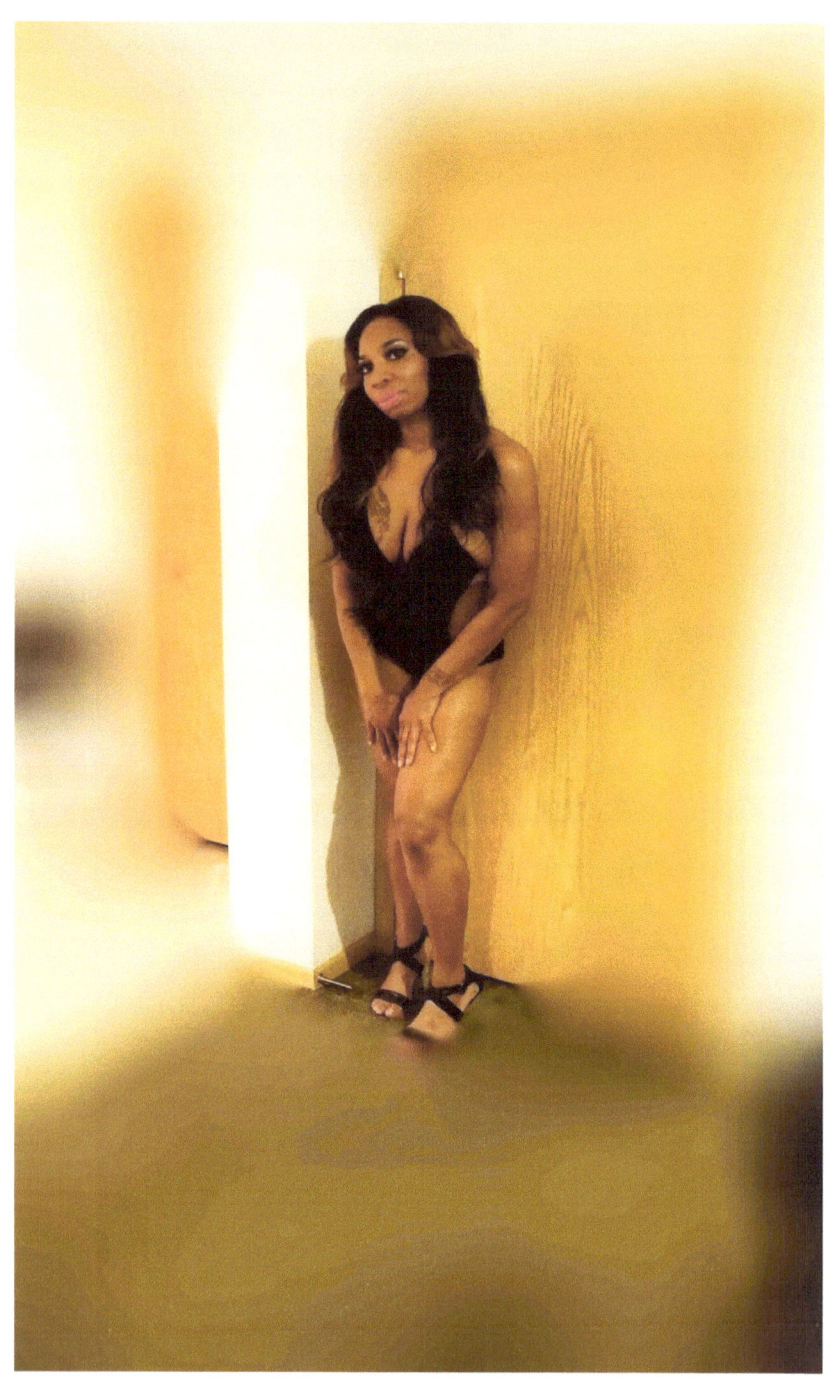

www.ingramcontent.com/pod-product-compliance
Lightning Source LLC
Chambersburg PA
CBHW050856290526
45792CB00002B/613